TWO YEARS WITHOUT SLEEP

Working Moms Talk about Having a Baby and a Job

Edited by Cathy Feldman

BPB

Blue Point Books

Also from Cathy Feldman
Published by Blue Point Books

THE MEN AT THE OFFICE
Working Women Talk About Working With Men

I WORK TOO
Working Talk About Their Dual-Career Lives

Library of Congress Catalog Card Number: 92-75762

ISBN 1-883423-01-5

Editor's Note:
All quotes not footnoted are from my interviews. A few of the women quoted asked me not to use their real names.

INTRODUCTION

Two Years Without Sleep is the first in a series of books I'm publishing based on over a year's interviews with women in business. Working moms said again and again that nobody ever told them what it was really like juggling a baby and a job.

I asked the women to tell me about their experiences and what they thought was important for other working moms to know. Their answers gave me this book. All I've had to do was quote them. I've paralleled their quotes with facts, information, and advice from experts to put the situations in perspective, but the women's stories, told in their own words, are the heart of the book.

The many women who talked so freely to me about their experiences share the hope that it will be a contribution to solving our problems in the work place. The more we learn to understand each other, the better our chances will be to build a better future for us all.

I thank the women who are making this series of books possible, and dedicate these books to them.

CF

TABLE OF CONTENTS

The Interviews

MARSHA BAILEY, Exec. Dir., Women's Economic Ventures
ELIOT BERTHA, Program Director, YMCA
MARYANN CORRENTI, Partner, Arthur Andersen & Co., Dallas
PENNY DAVIES, owner, Earthling Bookstore
NANCY DELUCIA, radio disk jockey
JANET ELLIS,* Partner in accounting firm
TERESA ELONSO,* M.D., Obstetrics and Gynecology
SARAH FENSTERMAKER, Professor of Sociology and Women's
    Studies, University of California, Santa Barbara
STINA HANS, CEO and owner, MCBA Software
JANE HONIKMAN, Executive Director, Postpartum Support
    International
STEPHANIE JAMES, Graphic Designer
VIRGINIA JONES,* resource planner in state government
BEVERLY KING, Program Administrator, Childcare Resource
    & Referral Program
CAROL LEWIS,* Partner in a law firm
MARTHA NORRIS,* Psychiatrist
JOANNE PARKS,* Business planner
IDA POINTER-GOMEZ, Loan Officer, Mid-State Bank
VIVIANNE POTTER, Business Manager, Whitney Associates
MARCIA ROSS,* photography teacher
SUSAN SANTANA, secretary at high tech company
KATHRYN SHAW, owner, Medical Billing Auditors
SALLY TASSANI, CEO, Tassani Communications
SUSAN TEW, Assistant Director Communications, Alan
    Guttmacher Institute
LINDA VASQUEZ, Licensed Insurance Agent
MARILYN WEIXEL, Vice-President Human Resources,
    Associate Group Insurance Administrators
ALISON WINTER, President, Northern Trust of California

* Not their real names. See Appendix A for list of other sources

PREGNANT AND
WORKING

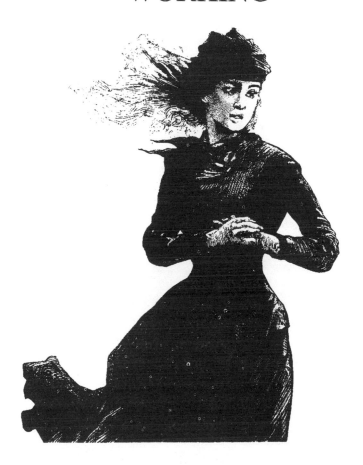

WOMEN IN THE WORKFORCE HAVING BABIES

80% of the women in the workforce in 1997 were of childbearing age.

89% of those women are expected to become pregnant during their working years. [1]

BABIES BORN IN THE UNITED STATES

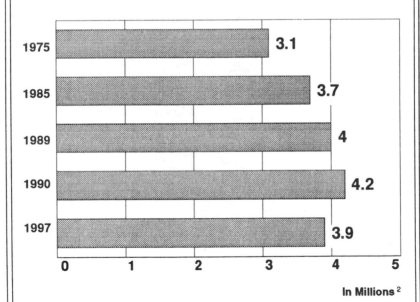

Year	(In Millions)
1975	3.1
1985	3.7
1989	4
1990	4.2
1997	3.9

In Millions [2]

1. Women's Legal Defense Fund base on statistics from the Census Bureau
2. National Center of Health Statistics

"In addition to my husband, I talked about having a baby with seven men in the office. I told them in advance that I wanted to have children, and if I did, how I wanted to handle it workwise.

"It was easy enough for them to sit there and say yes. Then I conceived two weeks after I mentioned it.

"When I announced I was pregnant, I can still remember the shocked look on the face of one of the men. It seemed to him that it had just been a thought.

"When the reality came, they said, 'Well this isn't exactly what we had in mind,' or 'Maybe we said yes, but we didn't know you really meant now.'"

— *Janet Ellis*

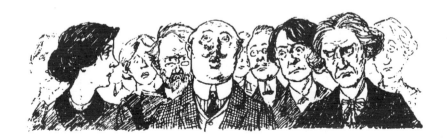

TELLING THE BOSS

TELL THE BOSS FIRST

The boss should be the first person in the organization to know you're pregnant. Confide in just a few friends in the office, and the boss will hear it second-hand and wonder if you're going to be straight about this. The boss's big fear is that you won't come back after having the baby even though you have agreed to.[1]

WHEN TO TELL THEM

Conventional wisdom holds you should announce your pregnancy sometime after your first trimester when you are past the point when the risk of miscarriage is the highest but before your waistline starts to show.

• Tune your schedule of announcing your pregnancy to suit your company.

HOW TO TELL THEM

• Present your pregnancy to your boss like any other business problem—with a solution attached.

• Don't try to get into specifics when you first tell the boss. Schedule a formal meeting to go over the details of your maternity leave.

• Be sure to know what your company's policies are both on paper and what they have done in the past with other employees.[2]

---

1. Walter Kiechel Jr., "A Guide for the Expectant Executive", *Fortune*, September 9, 1991
2. Diane Harris, "Maternity Leave Yours, Maternity Leave Hers", *Working Woman*, August 1991

"I delayed telling my partners that I was
pregnant until I couldn't hide it any
longer. I kept wearing looser clothes. Finally I
told them. Some of them were not happy.**"**

— *Carol Lewis*

"I approached my partners, three men, to tell
them I was thinking about starting a
family. One of them was difficult. He wanted
me to postpone it a year. I told him, 'Things
don't work out like that.' It turned out his
wife was pregnant and he wanted to take some
time off. I got no support or sympathy from
him the whole time I was pregnant.

"I've had to face the issue from the
employer's side as well. One of my employees
just got pregnant. Sure I invested a lot of time
and money training her. Yes, I worry about
what I'm going to go through replacing her
and starting all over again. But when she told
me, the first thing I said to her was,
'Congratulations. I'm happy for you.' She was
afraid to tell me. We talked about her coming
back. She really wants to, but she has a
one-year-old. I told her, 'You want to come
back, your job will be here.' A male colleague
told me that I didn't have to hold the job for
her legally. But she's great, and I hope she
will.**"**

— *Teresa Elonso*

PREGNANCY DISCRIMINATION ACT OF 1978*

Employers of 15 or more workers cannot:
- fire an employee because she is pregnant
- refuse an employee a promotion because she is pregnant
- force a woman to take pregnancy leave

Federal laws do not apply to claims of pregnancy discrimination in companies with 14 or fewer employees.[1]

FAMILY AND MEDICAL LEAVE ACT OF 1993*

Employers of 50 or more workers employed at least 20 weeks a year at or within 75 miles of an employee's work place must provide the worker who has been employed by that company at least 12 months the right to:
- up to 12 weeks of unpaid family leave in any 12 month period
- the same or equivalent job restored with equivalent benefits on return from leave [2]

WHAT TO DO TO PRESERVE YOUR JOB

No matter what size company you work for, find out what your company's leave policy is, try to arrange a mutually agreeable plan with your employer, and try to get what you're promised in writing. If that fails, work internally by talking to your human resources or personnel person or even your CEO. If you cannot reach an agreement, you can seek outside help through the EEOC's local office or your state's employment agency, but if you can stop these problems before they start, you will save yourself a lot of anguish.[3]

---

*These very general summaries of the laws should not be relied on as legal advice. Ed.
1. Abby J. Leibman, Executive Director, California Women's Law Center.
2. Facts on Working Women, Women's Bureau, U.S. Department of Labor, No. 93-1, March 1993. See Appendix B for more information on the Family Leave Act.
3. Helen Norton, Women's Legal Defense Fund. See the white pages of your phonebook under U.S. Government for your nearest Equal Employment Opportunity Commission (EEOC) office.

"I worked for my boss for about two and half years. I distinctly remember in our interview he asked me if I planned on having any more children. I said, 'You can't ask that.' Because I had taken classes and knew he couldn't. He said, 'You don't have to answer it, but it is a small business and I'd like to know where you're at.' My son was four at the time, so I told him, 'At this time, I have no distinct plans. But I don't know about the future.'

"I'm very loyal and he appreciated it. He gave me raises, promoted me to office manager. I made his business my life as much as I could. He was very good to me.

"When my son went into kindergarten, I decided to get off the pill. I didn't say anything to my boss because I didn't feel it was any of his business. I got pregnant two months later.

"I told him when I was six weeks pregnant. I was fair and upfront with him. He had an ad in the paper the next week. He said he didn't know if I'd have problems with my pregnancy so they wanted to start interviewing.

"They demoted me from being office manager. He took me out to lunch and said, 'Now that you're going to be leaving. . .'

"I said, 'I don't want to leave. I'm hoping we can work something out so that I can come back part time until I can come back full time.'

"I thought he would work with me. Instead he told me he didn't want to pay me commissions any more, just a base salary because they didn't want me selling any more. He wanted the clients to get used to me not being there. I was three months pregnant.

"They hired someone, took away my desk and told me I had to train this person. I had to sit next to the desk of the person I was training. I wanted to hold on to the job because I knew I was going to have a Caesarean and I wanted to get state disability. So I took a lot of this.

"Then they wanted to reduce my salary by $500 a month. And they told me I couldn't talk about the baby at work or have any calls to or from my husband and son. So I quit. I cried the whole way home. The next day was Christmas Eve.

"My husband called them and told them we were going to talk to an attorney. My boss called me and asked me to come back at my old salary. I should have done something at that point, but instead I went back in January.

"When I went back I got the cold shoulder. I just trained the person they had hired. They gave me my old salary, but they totally restructured my position. They didn't want me to sell or answer the phone.

"They treated me different. They said it was because I was different because I was pregnant, that my work was different. I came in late one time and they bawled me out. It was like night and day from the way they treated me before I got pregnant.

"Before I left to have the baby, they had me sign a form saying that my job was not guaranteed if I stayed out more than three months. I didn't want to go back there anyway, so I signed it and I didn't go back."

— *Linda Vasquez*

"I knew I needed to be a partner before I had a child. I'd say that after the child came my billable hours were down about 20-25%. As an associate, that would have been real tough. I don't think I would ever have been made a partner if I had the child without being a partner.**"**

— *Carol Lewis*

"I waited until I was tenured before I had my baby. It was the only way I could be sure of my position.**"**

— *Sarah Fenstermaker*

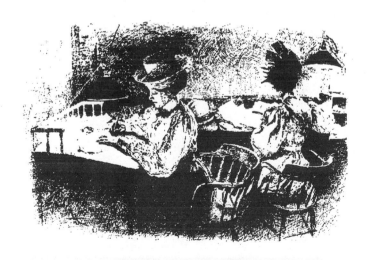

PROTECTING YOUR JOB

BEWARE THE OFFICE VULTURE

It doesn't matter how long you have been at your job, it doesn't matter how competent and well-liked you are, it doesn't matter how definite you have made your plans to return: It's still likely that some ambitious colleague will try to move in on your job.[1]

HOW TO PROTECT YOUR JOB ON MATERNITY LEAVE

Make the job easy for people filling it for you, but don't make it too easy. Limit your explanations to specific tasks that must be accomplished.[2]

- Arrange your leave with your boss and get it in writing
- Tell your co-workers carefully, making it clear you have a plan
- Reassign your duties by splitting them up among several people
- Inform your clients in writing and send copies to your boss
- Keep in touch by phone when you're gone
- Have office memos sent to you at home [3]

1. Pamela Redmond Satran, "How to Protect Your Job While On Maternity Leave", Copley News Service, March 3, 1991
2. Diane Harris, "Maternity Leave Yours, Maternity Leave Hers", *Working Women*, August 1991
3. Advice from authors Jean Marzollo and Marcie Schorr Hirsch in "Protecting Your Power Base When You're on Maternity Leave," *Working Women*, June 1990

"One of the reasons I didn't have children at a younger age was I was worried about building a career here. Now I realize a lot of this was my perception, because there were so few women above me. Would they perceive me as not being committed? Then I realized when I got to be 36, I had to do both. I had my first child at 36 in 1988, my second child at 38. In between I was made a partner in the firm.

"I remember coming back from maternity leave and questioning one of the partners I was close to, 'What did the partners think because I took three months off? Was there ever a doubt in their mind I wasn't coming back? Did they think I was any less committed?'

"He said, 'Maryann, everybody knows you. They know what a hard worker you are. They know how committed you are. It was never brought up. It was never an issue.' Which shows it was more in my mind than in theirs.

"I'm realizing today all you have to do is ask. Once you have made a name for yourself, established your credibility with a company, worked there 2 or 3 years, most companies say 'I will do anything to keep Sue or Mary. I'll take her 50% of the time rather than lose her.'"

— *Maryann Correnti*

Treatise on The Science and Practice of Midwifery

W. S. Playfair, M.D., 1876

Sympathetic Disturbances

"Shortly after conception various sympathetic disturbances of the system occur, and it is only very exceptionally that these are not established. They are generally most developed in women of highly nervous temperament; and they are, therefore, most marked in patients in the upper classes of society, in whom this class of organization is most common. Amongst the most frequent of these are various disorders of the gastro-intestinal canal . . . popularly known as the 'morning sickness.'"

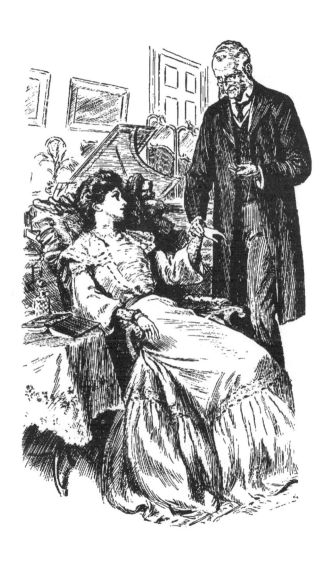

MORNING SICKNESS

WHAT IS MORNING SICKNESS?

"Morning sickness" is a term used to describe nausea and vomiting associated with early pregnancy. These symptoms occur in 60-80% of all pregnancies, and usually begin within six to eight weeks after the last menstrual period. They usually disappear or decrease dramatically near the end of the first trimester.

Current theories suggest the symptoms may be a result of neuro-chemical changes.

For many women, nausea and vomiting may be accompanied by other symptoms, including an aversion to certain smells like coffee or cigarette smoke. Other women are bothered by the sight of certain foods.

WHAT TO DO ABOUT IT

• Keep crackers by your bed. Eat one or two on waking, wait 15 minutes to get up
• Eat frequent small snacks or small meals
• Try to drink plenty of fluids. Drinking small amounts of liquids frequently may be easier than drinking a whole glass at once
• Heartburn may be contributing to your nausea. Most women find an antacid helps
• Try to minimize stress and increase rest periods
• If persistant and severe vomiting occurs several times a day, see your doctor.[1]

---

1. Paula Adams Hillard, "Coping With Morning Sickness", *Parents Magazine*, August 1990

"When I got pregnant, I was sick a lot. I wasn't out of work, but I felt so lousy I was probably only 75% of what I normally am. For the most part my work got done. Perhaps not in quite as timely a manner as it would have, but my boss was very understanding in letting me rearrange my schedule to fit my health.

"I don't deal well with feeling sick. I can deal with pain. But that general feeling of malaise just sort of undoes me. But it only lasted about three months. I worked until about a week before she was born."

— *Vivianne Potter*

"I had some morning sickness. I kept a glass of water next to me all the time to make sure the stuff was going down the right way. Every once in a while, more once in a while than I'd like to admit, I was sick. I drank a ton of water, more water than I ever had in my life. I lost it a few times, but I was very fortunate, I always made it to the bathroom. And I was very fortunate that nobody was ever in there so no one knew."

— *Carol Lewis*

THE WEIGHT THING

HOW MUCH WEIGHT SHOULD YOU GAIN

Weight gain is usually 3 to 5 pounds during first trimester. Most weight gain should occur during last three months, at the rate of about a pound a week.

- Average total weight gain—24 to 28 pounds.
- For underweight women—30 to 35 pounds.

It is a fallacy to believe a woman needs to eat twice as much food when she is pregnant. The basic rule is a pregnant woman should consume 300 extra calories a day.[1]

HOW TO CONTROL YOUR WEIGHT

- Keep a "safe house." Don't keep sweets around. If you have a craving to eat ice cream, make yourself go and get it.
- Try to get some exercise every day—walking, swimming, bike riding are all good for you.
- Eat your carbohydrates later in the day. It's almost best to exchange your breakfast with your dinner, i.e., eat protein in the morning and after noon.
- Have small frequent meals. It's normal to be hungry all the time when you're pregnant. If you eat a small amount every 2-4 hours, you won't overeat.
- Don't drink fruit juices but do drink plenty of water. Eat the fruit itself. That avoids the sugar "rush" from fruit juice.
- Consult your doctor before making any changes in your diet.[2]

---

1. National Institute of Medicine, 1990 recommendations
2. Elizabeth Toro, M.D., Obstetrics and Gynecology

"When you go to the doctor, they say to gain 25 to 35 pounds. 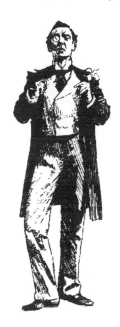 Every woman I've talked to has minimally gained forty. I had a real hard time with my OB. I felt like I was going into a weight loss clinic every time.

"I have a weight problem anyway, and I have to work out and really watch what I eat to maintain any kind of normalcy. Every time I went to him I was just totally guilted out. He told me I had a psychological problem.

"I had a friend he told the same thing to, then referred her to his wife, who's a psychologist."

—*Nancy DeLucia*

66 **I** went through three pregnancies. If I was negotiating a contract with someone and I was nine months pregnant, it was hard for them not to notice I was pregnant, since I gained 70 pounds each time. 99

— *Stina Hans*

66 **M** y son was nine and a half pounds when he was born. People in the office wanted me to go home. It kind of hurt for them to look at me. When I sat down, you'd never believe I could get up. That part was real fun. 99

— *Janet Ellis*

66 **I** was afraid I wouldn't be able to sit at my desk. You never know how the child is going to grow. I honestly worried that I would have to sit too far away from my desk. Fortunately it worked out okay. 99

— *Carol Lewis*

"I had to quit a month earlier than I expected. I was so huge I couldn't bend over any more, and I couldn't sit for long periods of time."

— *Marsha Bailey*

"When I was pregnant, I felt really well. But I couldn't sit for more than an hour. The night before I delivered my son, I was in a meeting with a client. Fortunately, I knew him well. I said, 'Guys, carry on. I've just got to walk around this conference table a couple times.'"

— *Maryann Correnti*

STEREOTYPES AND PERCEPTION

"The sight of a pregnant woman acts as a visual cue, eliciting a whole host of associations and stereotypes. People don't intend to discriminate against pregnant women."

— Jane Halpert, professor at
DePaul University [1]

"Part of the stereotype of women has to do with dependency, with notions that women are weak and work best in a supportive role rather than in a leadership position. If there are stereotypes about being a woman, they are tenfold about being a pregnant woman."

— Janet Spitz, management
professor at Rensseler
Polytechnic Institute [1]

"Assume that the perception is going to be that you are not the same productive, committed, aggressive worker you were before."

— Dawn D. Bennett-Alexander,
business professor, University of
Georgia [1]

"Most businesses function as a kind of family. When a woman is pregnant, her relationship with this family changes, arousing a whole range of emotions—including fears of abandonment. People without children may feel threatened. It's uncomfortable to have one's assumptions challenged."

— H. David Stein, professor of
psychiatry, Columbia-
Presbyterian Medical Center [2]

---

1. William Kiechel III, "A Guide for the Expectant Executive", *Fortune*, September 9, 1991.
2. Janice Kaplan, "Public Pregnancy", *Self*, April 1989

"**Y**ou really don't know how you want to react or how you want someone to react to you when you're pregnant. You enjoy the attention in a sense but at the same time you are always self-conscious."

— *Virginia Jackson*

"**W**hen you get pregnant, you are suddenly public property. People touch you. It's like your personal space is completely gone.

"People would come and touch my stomach. I'd think like, wait a minute! Their thumb was less than an inch from my pubic hair. If I wasn't pregnant, I would not feel comfortable with someone putting their thumb an inch from my pubic hair. People think it's totally okay if you're pregnant."

— *Stephanie James*

"**T**wo of the women I work with gave a shower for me and all the partners were invited. They gave me all the notes they got in response to the invitation. One of the male partners wrote, 'I'd love to come, but pregnant women make me nervous.' I never told him that I got it. It's funny but it's also kind of tragic."

— *Carol Lewis*

PREGNANT ON THE JOB

HOW LONG SHOULD YOU WORK?

Recommendations to how long you can keep working prior to your due date, if your doctor approves:

* Job that demands standing 4 hours a day or more: 24th week
* Job with physical activity: 28th week
* Job with little physical activity: as long as you feel well [1]

WORKING WHEN YOU'RE PREGNANT IS OKAY

In a study of pregnant medical residents who worked an average of 70 hours a week, it was found that the women were no more likely to have a miscarriage, stillbirth, tubal pregnancy, early delivery, or low-weight baby than a control group of women who worked only 35 hours a week.

The results suggest that a woman who takes care of herself and has a low risk pregnancy can work as much and as long as she wants.[2]

* If your work involves exposure to toxic substances like chemicals, certain metals, or X-rays known to affect the fetus, discuss your specific working conditions with your doctor to decide if it is safe for you to work while you're pregnant.[3]

---

1. Dr. Perri Klass, "Having Healthy Babies," *Cosmopolitan,* April 1992
2. A study by the National Institute of Health of 1,283 pregnant medical residents reported in *Working Woman,* September 1991
3. Sheldon H. Cherry, M.D., "On the Job and Pregnant," *Parents Magazine,* March 1991

"One of the woman in the firm was very concerned because I was going to work right up to the time I was going to have my child. She was concerned that my water might break. She didn't talk to me about this, but she had my secretary make sure that she had a blanket and things to clean things up in case it happened in the office. It had never occurred to me."

— Carol Lewis

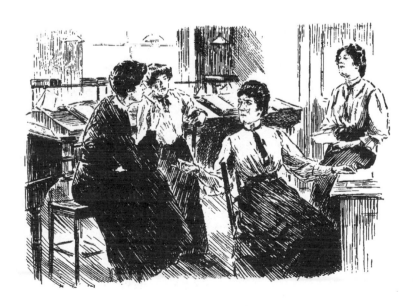

"I could have taken time off ahead of time, but I was really restless and working kept me busy. The day I delivered, I worked, I went to the doctor's office, went to the hospital, and had the baby that night. It took six hours."

—*Janet Ellis*

"Dorien was born on Christmas day of the first year we opened the new store. I worked until December 24. On December 25 I was home. It was the first day we had closed the store all year. I was making turkey and the water broke. I went to the hospital and had Dorien."

—*Penny Davies*

"The baby came ten days early. I had seen five clients that day. I went home at 5:40 and had the baby at 11:30. The next morning I was calling to leave my instructions with my secretary.

"I still remember thinking, the baby's here, and it's too soon. This pregnancy went by too fast. When you are a working mom, it goes by too fast. And when you're working up to the last minute, it goes even faster."

—*Carol Lewis*

THE BABY'S HERE!

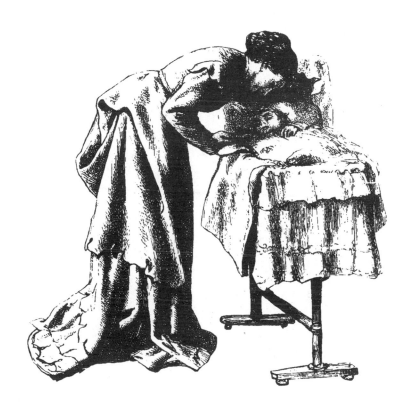

Treatise on The Science and Practice of Midwifery

W. S. Playfair, M.D., 1876

Prolonged Rest

"The most important part of the management of the puerperal state is the securing to the patient prolonged rest in the horizontal position, in order to favor proper involution of the uterus. For the first few days she should be kept as quiet and still as possible, not receiving the visits of any but her nearest relatives, thus avoiding all chances of undue excitement. It is customary among the better classes for the patient to remain in bed for eight or ten days; but, provided she be doing well, there can be no objection to her lying on the outside of the bed, or slipping on to a sofa, somewhat sooner. After ten days or a fortnight, she may be permitted to sit on a chair for a little."

"Y<!-- -->ou love your child, but at the same time you keep thinking, please go to sleep. Just the night before last, John woke up at 2 and wouldn't go back to bed until 5:30. I'd gone to bed at 11:30, so I only had two and a half hours of sleep.

"One day or two days is one thing. But when it goes on for a year, or two years, it's just unbelievable.

"Nobody ever told me when I had a baby and a job I'd have to go two years without sleep.

"You keep thinking this is the last time he'll do this. It doesn't happen."

— *Carol Lewis*

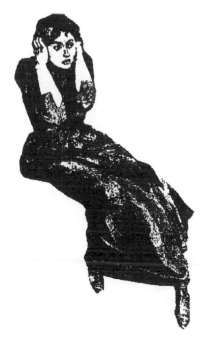

NEVER ENOUGH SLEEP

BABIES WAKE UP A LOT

Parents of newborns cannot expect a baby to have 8 uninterrupted hours of sleep.

* Newborns sleep randomly 16-18 hours a day, usually 2-4 hours at a time
* Sleeping through the night for an infant means sleeping without waking between 12 a.m. and 5 a.m.
* At age 1, infants sleep 13-14 hours a day [1]

THE EFFECTS OF SLEEP DEPRIVATION

* One night of not enough sleep affects mental concentration, flexibility and creativity
* Two nights of not enough sleep affects rote functioning
* Five days of sleep deprivation seriously impairs all functioning

Driving home on Friday is considered more dangerous than on Monday because so many people have been deprived of sleep during the work week. The U.S. Department of Transportation reports up to 200,000 traffic accidents may be sleep related. 20% of all drivers have dozed off at least once behind the wheel.[2]

---

1. A study of 60 first-time parent couples of newborns by Amy Wolfson, Patricia Lacks, Andrew Futterman, "Effects of Parent Training on Infant Sleep Patterns, Parents' Sress and Perceived Parental Confidence", *Journal of Consulting and Clinical Psychology*, February 1992.
2. Anastasia Toufexis, "Drowsy America", *Time*, December 17, 1990

"I have a sister-in-law whose child has been a lot more trouble than mine, and she said to me more than one time, 'You know in the war they use not allowing people to sleep as a torture.'"

— *Carol Lewis*

"For the first three months I sat in my bathrobe and I cried a lot because she didn't sleep. She would wake up every hour and a half and it would take her two hours to go through a four ounce bottle."

— *Stephanie James*

"A lot of people told me I wasn't going to be able to sleep, but there was no way I could comprehend what I was being told. A lot of people said, it's going to change your life. But we never really know how much."

— *Virginia Jones*

MOST WOMEN AREN'T READY

MANY FEEL ISOLATED

We found that women are prepared for childbirth, but no one prepared us for parenthood. It's likely that your mother is thousands of miles away. We no longer have the clan, the extended family, the built-in support groups to help the new mother. Now she's alone. She comes home with her new baby and she's on her own and expected to handle it all. She feels isolated and afraid. A lot of women can't cope.[1]

IT'S NOT WHAT YOU EXPECTED

Only one in four women view the role of mother with any semblance of realism beforehand. About 70% thought it would be "like playing house." Others imagined perfection—perfect mother, perfect children, perfect family.

The desire to have a child was based less on wanting to nurture than a wish to be nurtured. Women want children to love but primarily they want someone to love them back.

Some women feel isolated, others feel that their identities are being swallowed up by the baby.

Three out of four women resent their husbands' lack of practical and emotional support.[2]

---

1. Jane Honikman, Postpartum Support International
2. "The Motherhood Report: How Women Feel About Being Mothers", Lou Genevie and Eva Margolies, a survey of 1,100 American women between the ages of 18 and 80 in 1986-87.

"My baby was only five and a half pounds when she was born. Until she got up to eleven or twelve, which essentially was three months, she was waking up every two or three hours. It's only really been in the last several weeks that I've started to get my memory back. It's amazing what sleep deprivation really does. I have a friend who described it as the CRS syndrome. Can't Remember Stuff. She of course used the vernacular. 'Can't Remember Shit.' You just can't remember anything."

— *Susan Tew*

WHAT TO DO WHEN YOUR INFANT WAKES

- Realize that infants do not always need parents to help them return to sleep
- It is not always necessary to hold or nurse infant to sleep
- Gradually encourage infant to sleep at night by not allowing long daytime sleep, darkening bedroom at night but not during day, playing during daytime
- Establish a nighttime "focal" feeding between 10 and midnight
- Lengthen time before removing an awake and fussing baby from crib

Sleeping through night means sleeping consistently between 12 a.m. and 5 a.m., which an infant is generally able to do around 2 months.[1]

WHAT TO DO WHEN YOUR 2-YEAR-OLD WAKES

- Hold him until he's calm, then lay him back down
- Stay with him a few minutes
- Talk to him while patting his back
- Try not to create pattern of taking him out of bed

The baby should be comforted, encouraged to go back to sleep but not picked up. When you leave the room, he will probably cry. Come back in ten minutes and repeat the process. It may take him days to understand the new routine but he will.[2]

---

1. Amy Wolfson, Patricia Lacks, Andrew Futterman, "Effects of Parent Training on Infant Sleep Patterns, Parents' Sress and Perceived Parental Confidence", *Journal of Consulting and Clinical Psychology*, February 1992.
2. Bernice Weissbourd, "Getting a Good Night's Sleep", *Parents Magazine*, March 1991.

"My first baby started sleeping through the night on her 19th day. I think they must know when your patience has run out.

"She'd been up all night off and on, and nothing made any difference. I was rocking her in a chair and she was crying and crying. Finally, I had one of these Playtex bottles, with the little plastic liner, and I . . . Now I never lose my temper, and I certainly have never thrown anything in my life. But I took this bottle and threw it. The thing broke and formula was everywhere. It was on the ceiling, the walls, the carpet. There was formula dripping every place. The thing exploded when I threw it.

"My husband came in and said, 'What happened?' I said, 'I dropped her bottle.'

"Of course, I couldn't have dropped it. This thing was a bomb. So he delivered some roses to me that afternoon, and she slept through the night that night. So I think she got the message."

—Alison Winter

TAKING YOUR BABY TO BED

Some parents prefer to have their infants sleep with them in their bed and follow the advice of Dr. William Sears, a pediatrician in California.

"You cannot train a three-year-old baby like you do a pet. To teach a parent to just put their baby in a crib is wrong. What that baby learns is that the cage that I put him in is a fearful place to be. That sleep is not a pleasant state to enter. That when I wake up, there was no one there to help me. I think that can create mistrust within the baby.

"The fear that children will become overly dependent on their parents is unfounded. Children do leave the parents' bed. Between three and four there is a natural independency that children start wanting their own room.

"By bringing the child to your bed, you are teaching the baby intimacy. The children who have the style of nighttime parenting that I advocate for these parents, they learn intimacy."[1]

---

1. Dr. William Sears, author of "Nighttime Parenting", interviewed on *20/20*, August 28, 1992

"My baby's two and he still isn't sleeping through the night. Right now we're going through a separation problem. He's decided he's in love with me and John, and he doesn't want to be away from us. He cries when one of us leaves the room. Now he wakes up, calling for us, and he's all ready. He's standing up in the crib and has two blankets, one under each arm, ready to get into bed with us. I'm sure he'll outgrow it, but for now we just all go back to bed."

— *Martha Norris*

POSTPARTUM BLUES

WHAT TO EXPECT POSTPARTUM

Hormones can play a big role in postpartum blues. Levels of estrogen and progesterone plummet after birth; this dramatic change may trigger depression. The exhaustion and discomfort you may be feeling—from an episiotomy, uterine cramps, hemorrhoids, or breast engorgement—can contribute to feeling down.

- Allow yourself to feel bad
- Vent your feelings with friend who's had a baby
- Blues usually pass in ten days or so
- If blues persist, see your doctor to make sure it's not a medical problem. If it's not, ask for help from spouse, friends, and/or counselors.[1]

IF THE BLUES DON'T GO AWAY

Some women become clinically depressed postpartum. Signs of this depression are:

- Insomnia
- Agitation
- Feeling of worthlessness
- Decreased appetite
- Loss of interest in surroundings and in the baby

This kind of clinical depression requires counseling and possibly medication. If you have these symptoms and they do not go away, seek help from your doctor.[2]

---

1. Sheldon H. Cherry, M.D., "After the Baby is Born", *Parents Magazine*, December 1991
2. Dr. Lori Altshuler in "Factors Linked to Postpartum Depression", *Los Angeles Times*, November 27, 1990

"I did one project at home, a newsletter, and it just about drove me crazy. I was still too much in the throes of that postpartum stuff. The twins didn't sleep a lot. I mean they slept, but they never slept at the same time. So there was always one awake.

"Hormones are so weird. At the beginning I could not stand to hear them cry. It drove me nuts. Not in a bad way. It just made me terribly anxious whenever they cried.

"I was trying to work at the computer, then a baby starts crying. It seemed to me a horrible conflict, should I let the baby cry for few minutes and finish this, or should I drop this and go pick up the baby. That became this earthshaking decision."

— *Marsha Bailey*

"I got pregnant in November, and we moved in January. I came up here and started my own business very much pregnant. I had one week maternity leave. None of my clients wanted me to work, but the computer sits here in the house and I look at it, and it goes, 'Work on me.' And you need money. So you go to work."

— *Kathy Shaw*

POSTPARTUM DEPRESSION

Ten percent of the population of women do have something that is more than just an emotional adjustment problem. Some of these women are clinically depressed. Some are hospitalized. Some commit suicide, some kill their children. I describe it as the myth of motherhood colliding with the stigma of mental illness. You can't really know what it feels like to be part of that ten percent unless you've felt it. Sure, there's all the exhaustion and being isolated and not having friends.

One of the problems with dealing with postpartum depression is as women we've done a disservice to one another as part of the feminist movement. It's been very much a case of women not acknowledging their hormones because that was taboo.

In reality we are not just talking about reproductive hormones, we're talking about biochemical changes that occur that affect the adrenal glands and go on and affect the neurotransmitters. That was language we didn't have until the middle of the 80s.

Right now all the focus is on the birth and the baby. There is no thought as to what is the woman going to go home to. Where is her support group? Nobody asks that question.[1]

---

1. Jane Honikman, Postpartum Support International

"I had a very strong postpartum depression that lasted almost six months. I was never at a point I couldn't perform. I was just emotionally drained, trying to care for my child and deal with the hostile environment at work. There is such a stigma attached to depression or any kind of psychological illness. The pediatrician was the one who spotted it. She said, 'I think you're very depressed.' I was in denial. I said, 'No, I'm just tired.' Then when I started crying twenty times a day, I knew it was more than my hormonal imbalance.

"So I went to the postpartum group. I was so embarrassed to go to the group and identify myself. But they really helped me. Now I can say, yes, I had a postpartum depression. But you'd be surprised that within the medical community, there are certain individuals who think it's not okay to admit that. I was told by another female physician that I should never have shared that with anybody."

—*Teresa Elonso*

"I remember getting a call the day I got back home from the hospital. It's kind of funny. When I was in the office, first the guys were telling me not to work. But when they had something for me to do, they would give me a call and would be so grateful when I'd say yes. They'd say you really ought not to be doing it, but they kept calling. I should have said no, I couldn't because there was too much to be done and not enough hands to do it.

"I remember putting the baby down for a nap, knowing I had told a client who had called, I'd get back to him in 30 minutes. So I'm praying the child will go to sleep. The minute he was asleep, I literally bolted to the den, made the phone call and talked to the person. Then the baby started crying, and I had to try to cover it up and not to rush the client, but knowing I needed to get this over with. You bolt back to the baby and feed him. Back and forth like a ping pong ball.

"I had one client who loved to talk. He'd hear the baby cry and he'd say, 'It's good for the baby.' Here's the mom knowing the baby's hungry and needs to be fed. It was terrible."

— Carol Lewis

"We all know that at six weeks postpartum you can go back to work and you can have sex. That's what the medical community says. But ask the women. The majority of women probably are ready and are healed and probably can. But there are at least ten percent, and my guess is that it is probably a whole lot more, who aren't ready."

— Jane Honikman

"I went back to work when she was six weeks old. I had to. I didn't have a choice."

— Susan Santana

"Most don't have a choice any more. I went back when he was seven weeks old, by tacking on a week of vacation time. Some vacation."

— Nancy DeLucia

"The reality is you are postpartum for 21 years. Motherhood is a big job you've taken on."

— Jane Honikman

THERE ARE A LOT OF CHILDREN WITH WORKING MOMS

In 1992, about half of the 21 million children under age six in this country had mothers who held paying jobs. And 1997, nearly two-thirds of the 24.7 million children in this age group have mothers who are employed.[1]

Children Under 6 with Working Moms

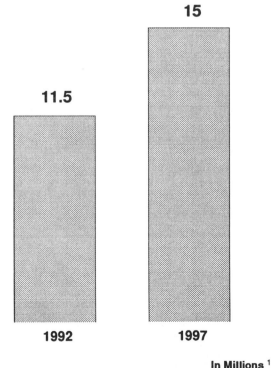

15

11.5

1992   1997

In Millions [1]

1 .Bureau of Labor Statistics

GOING BACK TO WORK

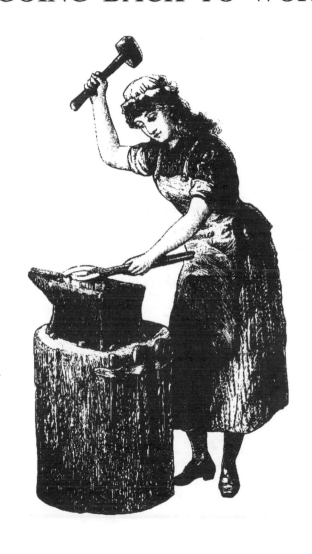

THERE ARE A LOT OF
WORKING MOMS

BETWEEN 1980 - 1997 THERE WAS A

+45% increase in total number of working women in the United States

+66% increase in total number of working women with children 2* or younger

IN 1997

3.5 million women returned to full-time jobs after having a baby [1]

WORKING WOMEN WITH NO CHILDREN AND BY AGE OF CHILDREN

In Thousands

	None	0-2*	3-5	6-17
1980	25,375	3,167	2,719	10,640
1997	34,969	5,252	4,442	13,894
% Increase	46%	66%	63%	31%

Bureau of Labor Statistics

1. Bureau of Labor Statistics
*35 months or younger

"When I went back to work, it was not hard. When I was at work, I did not even think about them. I did not anguish over leaving them. I was lucky. At that time I had in-home care. She was like their grandmother. She'd raised seven kids of her own. She was much more patient with them than I was.

"My feeling is, if you're going crazy at home, I don't believe that the person who births the baby is necessarily the only or the best person to take care of the baby. There are some people who are much better taking care of children; they are more skilled, more patient.

"I felt a little judgmentalism when my neighbor asked me how soon I went back to work. He's a doctor and his wife, a lawyer, had still not gone back to work after a year. He said, 'Boy, you were really brave to go back to work that early.' It didn't have anything to do with brave. It's just what I needed. If I was going to be going crazy when I was home with the twins, I'm not going to be a good parent. It means I'm going to be impatient. If I wanted to be a pre-school teacher, I'd do that. But I don't."

— Marsha Bailey

FOR SOME GOING BACK IS HARD

THREE FACTORS THAT CAN MAKE IT EASY OR HARD

* Quality of childcare
* What issues you've worked out with your husband and whether he lives up to the agreement
* Whether or not your work environment is supportive[1]

SOME NEED A TRANSITION PERIOD

Many women find they need a transition period to adjust to life as a working mother. In addition to the physical recovery process, there's an emotional impact. Don't be too ambitious about getting back in the swing professionally. Try to arrange a flexible schedule to ease back in.

The biggest worry about asking for a flexible arrangement is the concern that it will automatically shift your career into low gear. According to Ellen Klein, partner in the New York executive recruitment firm Scott-Bennett Inc., "You may be perceived as less serious; you will most likely move onto a slower track. Women should know that when they make that choice."

Managers sometimes equate hours spent in the office with professional dedication—to the detriment of working mothers.[2]

---

1. Lucia Gilbert, Ph.D. at University of Texas at Austin in "Easing Your Return to Work", *Parents Magazine*, June 1992
2. Diane Harris, "Maternity Leave Yours, Maternity Leave Hers", *Working Woman*, August 1991

"I went back to work after 8 weeks. There was a difference. When it was just me, I could handle stress. After I had my son, I blame it on those damn hormones, the stress was really hard. Especially feeling guilty about my son while I worked long hours, getting home late and leaving early, worrying about him.

"It really changed everything for me. It was almost like changed personalities. Maybe changed priorities might have been the theme. Little things set me off. Before I would just overlook it and go on. Now anything would set me off to the point I would think, what is wrong with me. Aren't the hormones right yet?"

—Ida Pointer-Gomez

A CASE FOR FLEX-TIME
THE AETNA STORY

In 1987 Aetna Life and Casualty found that nearly 33% of the 1,300 women who took maternity leave were not coming back to work at all. Managers rated the performance of women who did not return higher than those who did.

In 1988 they implemented a program offering up to six months unpaid family leave to its employees for births, adoptions, or serious illness in the family, in addition to the standard six weeks paid disability already in place. The employee's job was guaranteed, employee benefits continued, and the employee would work part time or from home based on a schedule worked out directly with the employee's manager.

- In 1988, 88% of new mothers returned
- In 1991, 91% of new mothers returned
- The length of family leave tended to be shorter than expected with most employees taking only two months
- 25% of women who returned said they had done so because the new leave program let them work part time or at home

Women who take maternity leave want to return to work, and they will be much more loyal and productive if their company is understanding about their personal lives.[1]

---

1. "Family Leave, without labor pains," Sherry Herchenroether, *Working Woman*, January 1992

""We have found that just implementing flexible work schedules is not enough. You need to have some sort of sensitivity training, gender-training; you have to have that awareness raised so male managers know why it is in the company's best interest to offer it. If you try to cram it down their throats, it's not going to be accepted. You have to have the people supervising having an understanding of it.

"But finally even some of the small companies have changed after the heads of the companies have had daughters who are out in the workplace. I was talking to the president of a small bank who told me, 'I did not think about alternative work schedules until my own daughter-in-law was working and she had a child. I realized we should be doing something like this.' ""

— Maryann Correnti

WRONG ASSUMPTIONS ABOUT FAMILY LEAVE

In a survey of 1,775 managers in a high tech company with offices throughout the United States it was found that most assumptions employers have about parental leave and productivity are wrong.

ASSUMPTION: Women give supervisors little notice of pregnancy or leave plans until far into their pregnancy.

REALITY: 73% of supervisors learned about impending leave in first 3 months of pregnancy.

ASSUMPTION: Women change their minds about when and if they return from leave.

REALITY: 68% employees followed through on original plans and 94% of women came back to work.

ASSUMPTION: Pregnant employees disrupt the office productivity.

REALITY: 82% of supervisors believed pregnancy did not affect the productivity of the employee and 93% believed it did not affect output of coworkers.

ASSUMPTION: While employees on leave, office productivity is disrupted.

REALITY: 52% of supervisors reported no difference in output of replacement compared to leave-taker, but 34% reported replacement did not perform as well as leave-taker.

MORE WRONG ASSUMPTIONS
ABOUT FAMILY LEAVE

ASSUMPTION: Productivity was disrupted when leave-taker returns.

REALITY: 73% of supervisors said returning employee was being 90% effective on job within 15 days of return.

ASSUMPTION: Supervisors and coworkers respond negatively to issue of parental leave.

REALITY: 77% of supervisors believed leave-taker's output was the same after return as before, while 16% reported an increase in productivity.

MOST MANAGERS WERE IN FAVOR OF PARENTAL LEAVE

75% of supervisors believed parental leave has positive effect on company's business and 77% were satisfied with how leave was handled.

Supervisors who had strong positive attitudes toward parental leave were twice as likely to be women than men. Lack of understanding of the company's leave policy was an important factor in negative attitudes held by some supervisors toward family leave. The study recommended that training be used to change this situation.[1]

---

1. "Parental Leave and Productivity: The Supervisor's View", Graham L. Staines and Ellen Galinsky. Families and Work Institute.

FAMILY LEAVE WORKS

FAMILY LEAVE IS CHEAPER

Worst case scenario study found that family leave was cheaper than replacing an employee
* It costs 32% of an employee's yearly salary to give them a parental leave.
* It costs between 75-150% of an employee's yearly salary to replace them.

The figures include the hidden costs, as reported by the supervisor: how much productivity was lost, how much the co-workers picked up and what their loss of productivity was. It is clear that parental leave costs an employer far less than replacing the employee.[1]

FAMILY LEAVE IS PRODUCTIVE

78% of women in highly accommodating companies, firms with paid parental leave polices, flexible schedule and supportive managers, returned to their jobs after childbirth, versus only half of those who worked for unaccommodating companies. Responsiveness paid off in higher productivity. Pregnant women in accommodating firms missed fewer days, were sick less often, worked longer into their pregnacies and were more likely to work beyond the hours for which they were paid.[2]

---

1. Rebecca Marra and Judith Linder, "The True Cost of Parental Leave." Families and Work Institute
2. "Accommodating Pregnancy in the Workplace, a study by National Council of Jewish Women

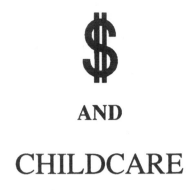

$

AND

CHILDCARE

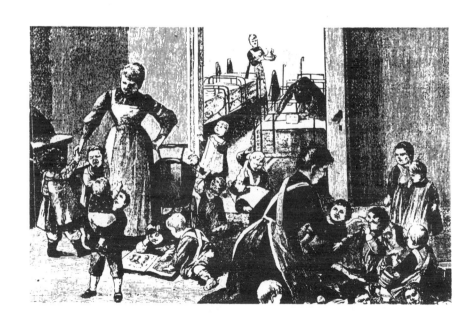

WHO'S GOING TO TAKE CARE
OF THE BABY?

84.9% of mothers between ages 23-31 rely on an individual to provide care for their infant.

96.3% of mothers between ages 29-39 rely on an individual to provide care for their infant.

Many childcare centers do not accept children under the age of three or accept them only at a higher fee. Most women rely on relatives to take care of their infants, often the father.

Mothers in low income families are more likely to lose their jobs because they can't find adequate childcare arrangements while mothers in high-income families are more likely to take time off work to handle childcare problems.[1]

65% of working mothers with infants reported trouble finding childcare, which affected their decision to return to work.[2]

Unless mothers get free babysitting from relatives, childcare costs are comparable to housing and taxes in terms of the bite they take out of the family budget.[3]

---

1. "Childcare: arrangements and costs", Jonathan R. Veum and Philip M. Gleason, Monthly Labor Review, October 1991. Statistics from 1983 and 1988 National Longitudinal Study for the Office of Economic Research, Bureau of Labor Statistics.
2. Children's Defense Fund
3. Families and Work Institute

"Childcare is expensive. I think it is the third largest chunk of what you are going to be spending your money on. It's a surprise for some parents. They don't expect it to cost that much. Here home childcare is $100 a week or more. In an infant center, the least expensive is $30 a day. In a family childcare home the cost averages between $100-110 in Santa Barbara area. It's lower in other states."

— Beverly King

"Childcare is probably one of the biggest problems. It's a heartwrenching decision as to what to do. There are a lot of alternatives but when you are working and trying to figure all that out, you don't have time. Going out and looking for the right place and interviewing all the right people. When you've got someone to help and you're happy with it, it's all great. When you haven't, it's a panic situation."

— Marcia Ross

BABIES COST A LOT

APPROXIMATE COST OF THE
FIRST YEAR OF YOUR BABY'S LIFE

Food	$1,250
Diapers	656
Clothes	546
Furniture	1,145
Bedding	256
Health care	645
Toys	349
Childcare*	**5,200**

*(based on national average for 40 weeks)

FIRST YEAR   **$10,047**[1]

EXPERTS ESTIMATE THE
SECOND YEAR COSTS A LITTLE MORE

SECOND YEAR   **$11.052**[2]

TOTAL
TWO YEARS $21,099

---

1. Rock-A-Buy Baby, American Demographics, January 1990; Expenditures on a Child by Families, 1997, Nutrition Policy Group, Agricultural Research Service, United States Department of Agriculture, 1997, and "Child care: arrangements and costs", Jonathan R. Veum and Philip M. Gleason, Monthly Labor Review, October 1991. (Adjusted for inflation - Ed.)
2. Expenditures on a Child by Families, 1997, Nutrition Policy Group, Agricultural Research Service, United States Department of Agriculture, 1997. This figure is the estimated annual expenditure for child born in 1997 to middle income ($33,500 - 59,700) husband and wife family. (Adjusted for inflation - Ed.)

"I wish I had known how much a baby was going to cost, and how much our needs get pushed aside before I'd had my baby. I didn't have a life for a year. I wish someone had told me that I wouldn't have a life."

— *Stephanie James*

"We can't really afford to have the baby. But if you keep waiting until you can afford it, you never will."

— *Susan Santana*

"I think financially it's more difficult when you are younger. We're more financially established the older we get, but physically we have a harder time. Sore arms, sore neck, physically it's more demanding when you're older. So you either pay with your dollars or your body."

— *Virginia Jones*

"There are the times when they can't go to daycare or they get sick or the daycare person gets sick and you are scrambling again to try to get a backup."

—*Marcia Ross*

"I've been really lucky. My supervisor is fifty. She's never had kids, but she's been married a long time. She's very understanding if I have to leave to take the baby to the doctor or whatever. Most of the other people who work under her are younger than her, and she's like a mother hen to us."

—*Susan Santana*

"One of the biggest problems is when the child is ill and the parent has to take off from work. Maybe the parent doesn't have any more sick days to take off.

"The state says that childcare centers can't keep a sick child. It's our policy at the infant center that a child can have one bowel movement which is loose, like diarrhea. But if there are two the same day, then the parent has to be notified to come pick up the child.

"Then there has to be a certain amount of time for the movement to be normal before they can bring the child back. The wellness and health issue is a difficult problem for most parents once they have a child in childcare. "
— *Beverly King*

"I went right back to work. Terry built a room where I could nurse the baby. Some bookstores had cats. I had a baby.

"About 6 or 7 months into Dorien being at the store, I realized that she was getting colds and flu because every customer in the store wanted to pick her up. I knew I couldn't keep her at the store so I put an ad in the paper and got a nanny. "
— *Penny Davies*

"Sometimes you just have to leave the baby with someone new. If you are desperate enough, if you have a deadline you have to meet and you are out of sick leave and you're out of vacation, you have to say, well, I'll just call three times an hour. "
— *Virginia Jones*

CHILDCARE AT WORK

1% of the nation's six million private establishments offer on-site childcare facilities

10% of private sector worksites with ten or more employees offer any childcare assistance

13% of all firms now offer flexible work schedules.

55% of the nation's big companies provide some form of childcare assistance.[1]

300 companies named managers addressing balancing work and family since 1990.

Time Warner set up a program that includes emergency childcare service in the employee's home when a child is ill or a regular baby sitter calls in sick. The program saves money by reducing the number of sick days employees take.[2]

Employer support for childcare reduces job turnover and childcare problems among working mothers with young children and can help employers address bottom line business concerns.[3]

---

1. Families and Work Institute
2. "Work-Family Programs Get Their Own Managers", Wall Street Journal, April 14, 1992
3. "Mothers in the Workplace", study by the National Council of Jewish Women

NANCY: I work with a lot of women. There are a lot of men there too, but there are a lot of the saleswomen at that station, and they are usually all decked out. When I take him to the office, they want to hold him, and I try to say, hold him this way, away from them. He's never gotten anybody yet. They say, "Don't worry about it," but I worry.

MARCIA: You always get spit up on.

STEPHANIE: I didn't wear silk for a year and a half.

VIRGINIA: I just took a bunch of clothes to the cleaners. They all had stains on the shoulder—food, spit up.

STEPHANIE: It used to be you just needed a extra pair of pantyhose in your desk. Now you need a change of clothes.

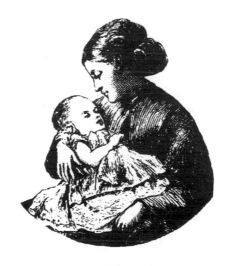

"Our company put in a plan called Section 125 which allows people to pay for eligible expenses with pre-tax rather than post-tax dollars. For dependent care, you can put in up to $5,000. My daughter's daycare is $7,500 a year. I save about $1,700 on the $5,000 that I can put into the plan.

"It costs our employees nothing. We pay the administrative fees. The money comes off of their gross pay so that it is never taxed. Not only does it save our employees money, but it actually saves us money, because we don't pay payroll taxes on it either, so whatever the administrative costs are, we actually save money. Last year we saved about $8,000, and we're just a small company."

— *Marilyn Weixel*

"The people at my place have been pretty supportive, but at the same time there is a definite line. If I do even talk about bringing him in, one of my supervisors, who has no children, says, 'You know, we have to be considerate of the other people in the office.'

"He's assuming that the child in the office will be a problem. I find that really annoying."

— *Virginia Jones*

"Even though I work at home, my kids go to daycare at least three times a week. I do that because I have to deal with insurance adjusters and attorneys. I can't sit here in a heavy negotiation and have them come running with 'Mommy, Mommy.'"

— *Kathy Shaw*

"The only time I brought my baby to work was when he was a week old. He slept while I was in the meeting.

"Then I took him in my office and was changing him, and he sprayed poop all over me. It was awful. My son loves this story, but it was certainly enough to make me not want to bring him around all the time."

— *Janet Ellis*

MILESTONES IN THE BABY'S FIRST YEAR

- 3-4 weeks: Baby able to focus on your face, turn toward your voice
- 2 months: Baby can smile in response to your smile, keep head up when held in sitting position, track objects with eyes, make sounds to express feelings
- 3-4 months: Baby can lift head up 90 degreees when on stomach, bring both hands together, laugh, roll from stomach to back, put everything in reaching distance in mouth, be fascinated exploring own hands and feet
- 5 months: Baby can sit alone briefly leaning on arms for support, do modified push-ups and make swimming motions, support weight when held under arms
- 6 months: Baby can sit independently, make consonant-vowel sounds, hold own bottle, support most of own weight when held in standing position
- 7-8 months: Baby can take sips from cup, start to crawl, pull up to standing position
- 9-10 months: Baby can crawl up stairs, say "mama" or "dada", take a few steps with support, feed himself finger food, respond to his name, stand with little support, sit down from standing position,
- 11 months: Baby can say long babbling sentences, drink independently from a cup, understand simple commands, take a few steps without support
- 12 months: Baby can walk with or without help, give a kiss on request, give and take a toy, imitate activities of adults and older siblings [1]

---

1. Dena K. Salmon, "First-Year Milestones", *Parents Magazine*, June 1992

WORKING AND
BREASTFEEDING

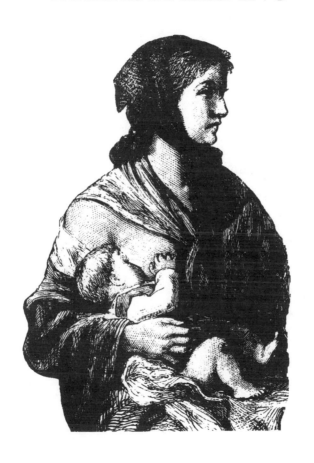

TO BREASTFEED OR NOT

7.1% mothers breastfed for at least 6 months in 1987

24% mothers breastfed for at least 6 months in 1997 [1]

PROS OF BREASTFEEDING

- Breastfeeding is an intimate way to connect with your baby
- Breast milk is superior to commercial formula because it contains antibodies that help protect your baby and keeps your baby healthier
- Breast milk is easier for most infants to digest
- Breast milk is free

PROS OF BOTTLEFEEDING

- Formula takes longer to digest, so babies sleep longer
- Easier to tell exactly how much baby is eating with bottles
- Bottlefeeding is easier in public

Many mothers combine breast- and bottlefeeding. Once breastfeeding is established, you can substitute a bottle of formula for breast milk once or twice a day. If your baby nurses the rest of the time, your milk supply will remain constant. [2]

---

1. La Leche League, 1997
2. Sheldon H. Cherry, M.D., "Deciding Whether to Breast-feed", *Parents Magazine*, September 1991

"I nursed the whole year. I made a commitment because I felt that was so important.

"I would nurse him in the morning, take him to the caregiver, work all morning, go there for lunch, nurse him, come back, work all afternoon, and pick him up or my husband would pick him up. I'd go home, nurse him before he went to bed and then come back to work. Or my husband would bring him here so I could nurse him if I had a meeting. It was constant juggling; it was awful."

— Eliot Bertha

"I'm still breast-feeding my son. The first half of the day before I can go see him I can stay pretty clean and nice. The second half of the day I'll come back and my blouse has banana on the shoulder, strawberry on the front. Our office is casual enough so that I don't even bother to change unless I have a meeting, in which case I do have a change of clothes."

— Virginia Jones

WEANING

HOW TO WEAN YOUR BABY

• If you plan to wean within first five months, introduce a bottle of breast milk or formula once a day when infant several weeks old
• If the baby breastfed exclusively for 3 or 4 months, it will be harder to wean
• Plan it to take a minimum of two weeks
• Substitute a bottle for the breast at one feeding
• Substitute the bottle again every three or four days
• Gradual changeover easier on both mother and baby
• Gradual changeover also lets breast-milk supply decrease slowly, preventing uncomfortable engorgement.[1]

HOW TO GET YOUR BABY TO TAKE A BOTTLE

• Get the baby acclimated to an artifical nipple
• Wait until baby is hungry and in good mood to introduce the bottle
• Try giving baby bottle before the breast. If the baby rejects it, try again the next time
• Have someone else give the baby the bottle, cuddling and talking during feeding as you usually do
• If you have to introduce the bottle, keep your breasts well-hidden.[2]

---

1. Katherine Karlsrud, M.D. with Dodi Schultz, "Weaning From the Breast", *Parents Magazine*, October 1991
2. Arlene Eisenberg, Heidi E. Murkoff, and Sandee E. Hathaway, "What to Expect the First Year", Workman Publishing

"Shortly after my son was born, I had a client meeting that was called for one o'clock. I nursed my son, then I went to the client's. It got to be three o'clock, four o'clock. And you know how men sometimes get long winded. I knew I'd only left one bottle of milk. The meeting was still going on. They knew I had come in from maternity leave. I finally said, "I'm really sorry, I have to reschedule for another day." You can't just leave a child at home with no milk. Nobody else could feed him. The milk machine was at the client's. It was very early in my maternity, so I hadn't built up my production yet. Later I was always sure to leave plenty of milk in the refrigerator."

— Maryann Correnti

"**I**'m still nursing my baby, he's only five months old. I have to pump at work, but I don't have a break. I don't have a lunch hour. I'm on the air and there is no leaving.

"So what I have to do is shut the venetian blinds. There are windows to the news studio and then we have an AM station down the hall and you can see right through, and then there's a window on the door.

"So every day I have to hang newspaper on two of the windows. My husband came down and installed a lock on the studio door. Then I plan when I'm going to pump when I go into 12 songs in a row. At ten away from the top of the hour I talk, I play two songs, I hit a jingle, then I have to play two songs again. So I have to pump within four songs. I'm doing the thing where I have the double, one on each side.

"I hang this little sign on the door that says, 'Please come back in ten minutes.' At first when I was doing it, everybody was going, 'What's she doing in there?' They're thinking I have some weird trick or I don't want anyone to talk to me or something. It's okay now. It's a pain, but it's worth it. You just get into the routine of it."

—*Nancy DeLucia*

"One of the things about working is when you work in an office, you don't have anywhere to go to pump other than a bathroom. If you go to an employee lounge, anybody can walk in. And in our case, we don't have one. I have to go into the bathroom and get semi-undressed and pump. I'd have the secretaries and other women walk in.

"It's funny to see other women's reactions. One of the women had nursed her son and expressed milk as well. She was completely nonchalant. She said, 'Hi, how are you doing. Boy, you sure get a lot fast.' Then the other two women who have not had kids were very embarrassed. One of them would avert her eyes and wash her hands and get out of the bathroom as quickly as she could."

— Virginia Jones

"There was one guy I worked with who kept making jokes, 'Nancy, is it true that you have pictures of missing children on the sides of your breasts?' It was funny at first, but he went on and on, and I had to tell him to shut up.

"I confronted him. I said, 'You know, it's not funny anymore. You're making me uncomfortable so will you stop.' He was shocked that I confronted him with it. I didn't yell at him or get mad. After I told him, I went into this other room and burst into tears.

"Then my boss, who's a woman, talked to him and said, 'You can't say anything and don't ignore her.' It was uncomfortable for a couple days. Now he still jokes around with me but he doesn't joke about my breasts. I don't think he knew it was bothering me."

— *Nancy DeLucia*

THE BABY OR THE JOB?

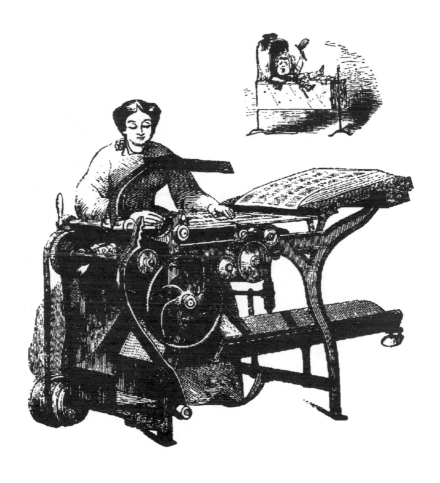

IS THE AMERICAN MOTHER HAPPY?

A Survey of 22,000 Women

49% were as happy before having baby as after

44% were happier after baby

7% were less happy after baby

53% would work even if didn't need money

80% wish could work only part time

71% pleased with childcare arrangements

53% love husband and children equally

43% husbands help with housework when asked

38% husbands share equally in child rearing

Both stay-at-home moms and working moms wish they had more time to spend with their kids.

The most stressful time of day for working moms is dinnertime.

The most stressful time of day for stay-at-home moms is kids' bedtime.[1]

---

1. Margery D. Rosen, "The American Mother, a landmark survey for the 1990s", *Ladies Home Journal*, May 1990.

"The corporate world still believes that women are only there to supplement the men's income. If they want to have children, they are not committed to their jobs.

"If you have a sick child and you stay home to take care of that child, you lose your job. If you leave that child home alone, you get thrown in jail. The barriers for working women are getting more insurmountable, especially since we live in a two-wage earner economy. A woman can't choose between her dignity and her job anymore. Her job has to win every time."

— *Barbara Otto*

"The climate of the workplace doesn't accommodate having a baby and a job. It's the rules that separate out as much as possible the personal needs of the worker from the workplace generally. You come to work to do your job the way we the employers say it will be done. That's true for coalminers as well as new moms."

— *Carol Lewis*

"When I went back to work there was a lot of stress. Before I had the baby, if I wanted to stay to 8 or 9 o'clock, there was no problem. Well, I could not afford to stay any longer. I had a baby sitter. I had to pick up a child by 5:30, regardless of what the traffic was.

"The people I worked with weren't sympathetic. They either had grown children or never had any children or didn't take care of their children. It became really stressful because they didn't want to know what my personal problems were. Their attitude was that I wasn't helping enough. But I felt that they just didn't have enough people to do the necessary work because they had been laying so many people off to save money, which was poor management.

"My husband was laid off from his job, but he found another one in Santa Barbara. The bank had tightened up on their employment so they weren't transferring people back in, and Santa Barbara is such a tight market anyway. So I left. I think they were happy to get rid of me. It was mutually agreed that it was nice for me to be leaving."

—*Ida Pointer-Gomez*

"The workplace treats having babies as personal problems. Everybody has their way of basically being in the closet about how awful they feel and about how poorly they are managing. One of the reasons they are in the closet is because we can't reveal the secret that we are incompetent at that moment. The work world is not arranged for that. Nobody understands and there are real sanctions if you appear not to be put together correctly.

"I wasn't telling everybody I was expressing milk after class before my office hours. Even that, even in these days, was asking too much of people. That's a problem with the way we organize work and the intersection of work and home. Personal problems simply do not exist. And if they do exist, they are not problems for the workplace problems. My baby was MY problem.

"You have to pretend so much. You have to pretend that you are blissfully happy, which is another thing that isn't always the case. You wouldn't give the baby back. On the other hand, it is the hardest thing you've ever done. People don't understand that, certainly people who haven't been through it."

— Sarah Fenstermaker

"If you look at the 80s, there was an attitude of employees saying: what can you do for me? Now I think the employer is saying, what can you do for me?

"I find we really have to look for people who are not only bright but have the right work ethic. Now the economy is not good. People are understanding that they really have to work more.

"In the 70s and 80s there was talk about a four day work week. Now I look at my people's time sheets on a monthly basis, and I'm really looking for them to work 40, 50 hours and up. If they aren't, I wonder about that employee, and we may have a problem."

— *Sally Tassani*

"I had to terminate an employee a little while ago because her attendance was abysmal. We didn't necessarily think that she was malingering. But either she was sick or her kid was sick. I felt terrible, but sometimes you have to draw the line. We probably bent over backwards a lot farther than most companies would. But we wouldn't be serving our other employees or customers if we didn't tell people there are certain limits."

— *Marilyn Weixel*

"When I had my first son, I would come in to work fifteen minutes late every day. It was always something like I'd pick him up and he'd throw up on me so I'd have to change. Jane, my boss, was really mad at me. She was really curt about it. She was all business, all professional. She said, 'Linda, I don't want to hear it any more. Get here by 9 o'clock.' I was getting no sympathy even from a woman. I always stayed late to make up for it, but I just couldn't get there on time.

"Then when she had her baby, I ran her office for her. She took off for a summer. When she came back she said, 'I'm really sorry. Now I know what you're going through.' She'd come in late because the baby threw up on her or she was up all night nursing."

— *Linda Vasquez*

"Our culture says that even if I'm not home, I'm still expected to carry out everything there. I'm a single mother, so I'm in deep trouble in terms of fulfilling the right picture. I saw this ad, a big come on from the phone company that says, 'Starting January 1, we will now be able to tell you a four hour period in which we will arrive to do maintenance on your home.' That's a big accommodation for them. But most women don't have the ability to sit around for four hours."

— *Sarah Fenstermaker*

"I feel less professional when I have to take her with me, even if it's just to run into a printshop and pick up an order. I can't leave her in the car. Number one it's against the law and number two I feel weird about leaving her there anyway. Even if it's right in front of the door. I feel kind of funny. I walk in and people say, 'Oh, you have your daughter with you today. How are you working?'"

— Stephanie James

"I had a situation where my mother-in-law had a meeting and the woman I took him to was really sick, so I had to bring him into work. Luckily I have a woman who is my superior, and she understood.

"I felt really weird. I felt guilty, like I shouldn't be bringing him here even though they just loved him. In a way I felt a little unprofessional."

— Nancy DeLucia

"When a father brings his children with him to a meeting, people say, 'Gee, what a good dad. He's interested in taking care of his children.' I just totally resent that. If I did that, the comment would be, 'What a poor professional.'"

— Janet Ellis

SOMETIMES PRIORITIES CHANGE

SOME WOULD RATHER STAY HOME

In a 1990 Roper poll, the 51% of working women with children under 13 would prefer to stay home rather than hold a paying job, while only 42% would rather work.

In 1985, 51% chose employment versus 45% who preferred homemaking.[1]

20% of women said their marriages improved after having a baby, 40% said they got worse.

50% of women felt cheated, that they were missing the best years of their kids' lives.[2]

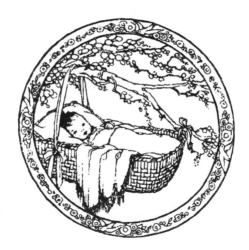

1. Peter Kerr, "Free Time Valued Over Money", *New York Times*, October 25, 1990

2. Lou Genevie and Eva Margolies, "The Motherhood Report: How Women Feel About Being Mothers", a survey of 1,100 American women between the ages of 18 and 80 in 1986-87.

"I'm leaving the department head position. I'm cutting back to 20 hours a week and I won't have the benefits or things I have as a full time executive.

"One of the things that made me make my decision to leave my position was that the caregiver for my son takes him to a park on Wednesdays when all the moms and their kids are there. I would go on Wednesdays and nurse him. One Wednesday Billy was so sad when I left, I remember my heart just tore.

"The other thing was he would never come to me. He would always go to the caregiver at the park. And that broke my heart. He was choosing her over me, and I said there is no way I will do this another year.

"I went home and said to my husband, 'This is my decision and we have to work this through because I cannot go on with it.'

"My husband is an insurance broker, and we've decided he'll have to increase his income by a certain amount in order to put me on his health plan. For me it's kind of unsettling, because I thought I always had to be able to provide for myself and make ends meet. Now I'm kind of giving up that control. I always thought we would share things and be more equal.

"When I made my decision to leave working full time, I felt like a whole burden had been lifted off me. I felt good even being able to talk to people because I felt like I wasn't hiding what was important to me. I think before I was afraid to say how I felt because I didn't want to hurt my job. Now I'm committed but I know what I've decided to do I'm going to do. But I can do 100% while I'm here because I know how it is going to be.

"The message that is put out is that you can do it all, you can have a career and have children. My whole attitude changed after I had my child. I can think of all the positives of working, and yet the deeper hurt that would come down the road isn't worth it. I think on my deathbed, what am I going to remember? That I wish I'd spent more time working or I wish I'd spent more time with my child?"

— *Eliot Bertha*

IT'S HARD TO BE AN OLD FASHIONED MAMA

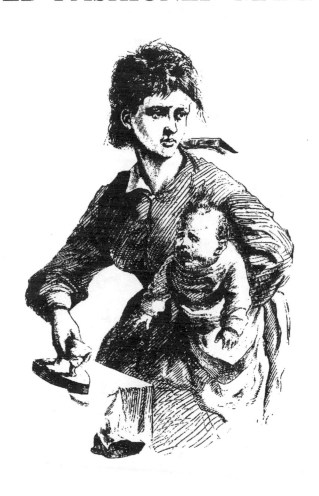

WHAT WOMEN THINK ABOUT MEN

A SURVEY OF 3000 WOMEN

In 1970, about 30% of women believed "Most men are basically selfish and self-centered." In 1990 more than 40% believed that statement was true.

In 1970, 70% of women believe "most men were basically kind, gentle and thoughtful." In 1990 only 50% of the women thought that statement was true.

Women were asked how satisfied they were with 15 different aspects of their lives in 1990:
• Top three: children, friends, husbands or other men in their lives
• Bottom two: job opportunities, income.[1]

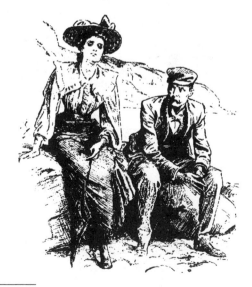

---

1. Virginia Slims surveys conducted by the Roper Organization cited in "Heavy Duty Anger", *Los Angeles Times*, September 23, 1990

"**M**y husband sees childcare as strictly the mom's role. He does the dishes and the laundry, everything else is up to me. I take them to childcare, I change the diapers, I potty train them. We fight a lot about that.

"I didn't breastfeed so feeding my baby at night didn't need me to do it. When he would start crying, my husband always pretended not to hear him so he wouldn't have to get up. He'd never help unless I actually forced him to. We'd play this game of both pretending to be asleep until I couldn't stand it any longer. By the time I had my second baby, he was an expert at it."

— *Joanne Parks*

"**M**y husband has always been very good about doing housework. We had a recent conversation. He was feeling put out like he was doing more than his share and I was doing less than my share. Then it came up that he didn't consider vacuuming and cleaning the bathroom as part of the equation. That was something he never did when he had his own place.

"All he was looking at was I didn't clean up the kitchen as much as he did. But I was cleaning the bathroom and vacuuming. Finally he realized he had to count bathrooms too."

— *Marsha Bailey*

"My husband wanted me to be a real true old fashioned mama. So I had to get him straight on that. I told him, 'Wait just a minute now. If I've got to work, and I've got to go this early and come home this late, I cannot do all the things you think I should be doing. You want me to get in bed by 9 o'clock? Good luck.'

"I played it through. I said, 'You want the dishes washed, you want the clothes washed, you want this all done, but don't tell me I have to go to bed at 9 o'clock. When I finished it, I'll be to bed.' It was like midnight when I got in bed. I did that for a couple nights and he realized that it could not be done. And he started helping. I knew I couldn't argue with him any more. He had to see it. I played the picture for him. After all, he gets home before I do, why can't he have dinner ready. Why couldn't he wash? I had to show him before he could realize it could not be done. Then he kicked in."

— *Ida Pointer-Gomez*

WILL I EVER GET BACK
IN SHAPE?

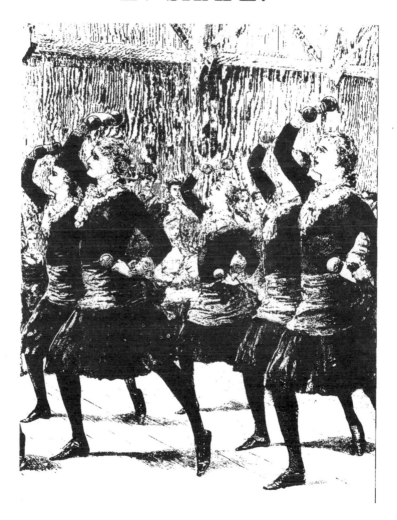

STEPHANIE: I ain't 34 perky any more.

VIRGINIA: You are supposed to have the baby, lose the weight, work, and do it all, and look like Demi Moore. I was determined not to worry about it. I wasn't going to worry about the weight gain. I wasn't to worry about the weight loss. But now it's starting to get to me, being out of shape.

SUSAN: I was the same way. I thought, I am who I am. If you like me for me, then that's great. If you don't like me for me, that's your problem, not my problem.

I think a lot of it is society. You look at all the TV ads and magazine. They are all these women who are size 2 or 3.

MARCIA: It's not just the ads. It's like movies and television where there are working mothers and women who have children, they're actresses who spend their whole life, like Cher or someone, working out. Cher works out ten hours a day. That's her life. That's what society sees. There are a lot of older women in the media who have children now, but they also spend all this time on their bodies. And we're out there trying to work and take care of the kids, and we don't have that kind of time to spend on our bodies.

STEPHANIE: I kind of feel like damaged goods. I feel like a man's not going to look at me, even if I'm wearing the same dress I wore a year and half ago, they're not going to look at me the same way. I feel like everything has shifted in such a way that I don't look like some hot young thing. I have a backless minidress I used to wear out dancing. I look at it now and say, this is ludicrous. I could never wear this.

WILL I EVER GET BACK IN SHAPE? • **93**

NANCY: A lot of it is putting pressure on yourself. You know, you're taking all these pictures of the baby. And I want pictures of me with the baby. I perceive myself smaller than I am. I see the pictures and go, my God!

MARCIA: I found that in a lot of my pictures the past year I looked tired, I look harried. I say who is that person. She looks so tired, frazzled. And this is how I'm going to be remembered!

WORKING MOMS WITH BABIES

41.9% of all women with infants 2* or younger worked in 1980.

55.4% of all women with infants 2* or younger worked in 1997.[1]

WORKING WOMEN WITH BABIES
2* AND UNDER
1975 - 1997

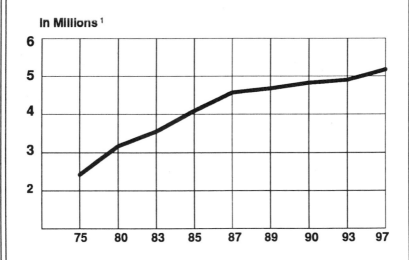

In Millions[1]

1. Bureau of Labor Statistics
*35 months or younger

MAKING IT WORK

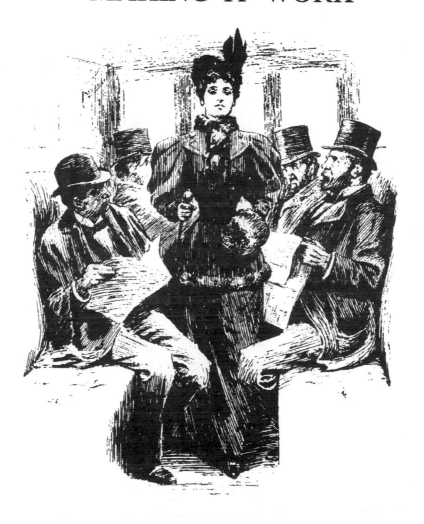

NEVER ENOUGH TIME

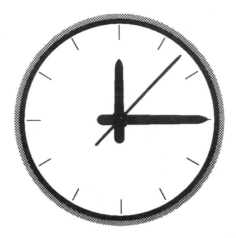

Americans are starved for time. Paid time off for vacations, sick leave, personal days, and holidays declined 15% in the 1980s. Americans are putting in an extra month of work a year.

If Americans continue to work at current rate, in 20 years they will be on the job for 60 hours a week, 50 weeks a year.[1]

Citizens of the European Community average between 25 and 30 days of paid vacation a year. Americans get less than half as many.[2]

The amount of "total contact time" between parents and children has dropped 40% over the past 25 years.[3]

---

1. Economists Laura Leete-Guy and Juliet B. Schor in a report for the Economic Policy Institute. "Nothing Leisurely About Time Off", *Los Angeles* Times, March 22, 1992.
2. Andrew Shapiro, "We're Number One!"
3. Family Research Council, Washington, D.C.

"When you're working, you have to be an expert at organization. My best advice is always to get up early because the mornings are awful. Everything takes longer getting the kids ready.

"I get up at 6:30 since I have to be at work at 8:30. My husband doesn't want to get up. The kids don't want to get up. And you're always having to rush them into the car to get them to childcare and end up doing 70 on the freeway to get to work on time.

"The trick is to save time anyway you can. One of the things I do is put on my makeup with one hand while I curl my hair with the other. It sounds dumb but it saves me time."

—Joanne Parks

IS THE MEDIA
BRAINWASHING YOU?

"Women all over the country are feeling inadequate trying to balance the responsiblities between home and work. No one feels like they have enough time, and almost unanimously they are worried over what they are doing to their children by not staying home with them.

"I'm very suspicious of the view of the bedraggled juggler. Why? Because jugglers who cope well are happy people. In fact, my research shows that if you want a happy home life, you need a significant involvement away from home.

"My findings show that women with jobs liked their home life better than women who stayed at home; and at the workplace, women and men who had families liked their jobs better than men and women who were single.

"If we confine ourselves to one role, no matter how pleasant it seems at first, we starve emotionally and psychologically.

"Everybody needs different sets of people in their lives. For a sense of wholeness as a human being, you need different parts. The juggler image says that if you have all these parts you will feel fragmented. The truth is that you need all these parts to feel whole."[1]

---

1. Faye Crosby, "Juggling: The Unexpected Advantages of Balancing Career and Home for Women and Their Families", in *Los Angeles Times*, October 22, 1991

VIRGINIA: The hardest thing about being a working mother is you have to let other things go, prioritize. There's never enough time.

SUSAN: There's never enough time for anything: grocery shopping, baths, showers.

NANCY: Taking a shower is a big one.

STEPHANIE: Eating. That's another big one. Think how wonderful it would be just to sit down to eat. I never get through an entire meal.

NANCY: I couldn't imagine what it would be like. I thought I'd have time to do everything. Before the baby I always went to the bank, went to my aerobics class, did my grocery shopping, and got stuff done at home. It was a great schedule for that.

I'd like to only work three days a week, that would be great, but I have to be there full time to get medical insurance.

"Only now when I'm meeting other working moms am I feeling less isolated. I felt, does anyone really know the emotions that I'm going through. I'd love to be able to go to the park and play with my kids, go to the zoo, but I can't afford it financially and timewise. These other women have taught me and reassured me that our children are learning to be self-supportive and self-sufficient, and they will survive."

— Kathy Shaw

"It's very hard for me to imagine just staying at home. Even if that was an option economically, I don't see that would be an option for my personal health. Raising a child is as stressful as working. And it's a very different kind of stress. When we have a long weekend or we take a vacation, I'm ready to go back to work because I need more grownup interaction. My mother had four kids in the span of six years, and she was a homemaker. Just having one child, I can't imagine having to deal with four of them all the time and not ever having any relief or going anywhere or doing anything else."

— Vivianne Potter

"I wish I hadn't waited so long to have the children. They bring so much joy to my life that I wish I could have worked a couple more in before I got too old. The children have brought a tremendous amount of balance into my life. Everybody needs to look at the birds again and trees again and bring yourself back to basics to make you a much more whole person."

— *Maryann Correnti*

"Before you could go wherever you wanted, do whatever you wanted without having to do the diaper bag and pack her up. But it's worth it because I look at her and she changes every day. And when she reaches up and says, 'Mama', you just melt."

— *Susan Santana*

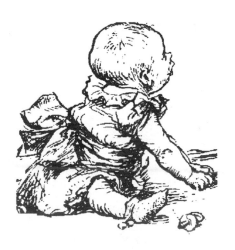

APPENDIX A

Included below are the names and address of some of the organizations helping working moms. Look in the Yellow Pages of your local phone book under Childcare for local and state agencies that act as referral centers. They can be a big help.

9to5, National Association of Working Women, 238 Wisconsin Ave., Milwaukee, WI 53203. (414)274-0925

9to5 Toll-Free Job Survival Hotline: (800)522-0925

California Women's Law Center, 6024 Wilshire Boulevard, Los Angeles, CA 90036. (213)935-4101

Children's Defense Fund, 122 C Street, N.W., Washington, D.C. 20001. (202)628-8787

Families and Work Institute, 330 Seventh Avenue, New York, NY 10001. (212)465-2044

La Leche League, 1101 Connecticut Avenue N.W., Washington, DC, 20036. (800)525-3243

ChildCare Aware: National Association of Child Care Resource and Referral Agencies (NACCRRA), 2116 Campus Drive SE, Rochester, MN 55904. (800)424-2246.

National Association for the Education of Young Children, 1834 Connecticut Avenue, N.W., Washington, DC 20009. (800)424-2460

Postpartum Educaton for Parents, P.O. Box 6154, Santa Barbara, CA 93160. (805)564-3888

Postpartum Support International, 927 North Kellogg Avenue, Santa Barbara, CA 93111. (805)967-7636

Women's Bureau, U.S. Department of Labor, 200 Constitution Ave, N.W., Washington, D.C. 20210. (800)827-5335. There are also regional offices in Atlanta, Boston, Chicago, Dallas, Denver, Kansas City, Philadelphia, San Francisco, and Seattle

Women Employed, 22 W. Monroe, Suite 1400, Chicago, IL 60603 (312)782-5249

APPENDIX B

SUMMARY
THE FAMILY AND MEDICAL LEAVE ACT OF 1993

Public and private sector employees who have been employed by the employer for one year and work at least 1,250 hours (25 hours a week) can take up to 12 weeks of unpaid leave in any 12 month period for: the birth or adoption of a child; acquiring a foster child; the serious illness of a child, spouse, or parent; and, the serious illness of the employee.

- The right to take leave applies equally to male and female workers of employers who employ 50 or more workers at least 20 weeks a year at or within 75 miles of the employee's workplace.

- Leave can be taken intermittently, is subject to employer approval, and does not result in a reduction in the total amount of leave to which the employee is entitled.

- When husband and wife work for the same employer, the total amount of leave that they may take is limited to 12 weeks if they are taking leave for the birth or adoption of a child or to care for a sick parent.

- An employee may elect or an employer may require the employee to substitute categories of paid leave for any part of the 12-week period.

- The employer maintains any pre-existing health insurance for the duration of the leave, at the level and under the same conditions coverage was provided prior to commencement of the leave.

- The employee must be restored to the original or an equivalent position with equivalent benefits, pay, and all other terms and conditions of employment.

- An employer may require certification from a health care provider to support a claim for leave.

- When the need for leave is foreseeable, an employee is required to provide at least 30 days advance notice.

- The highest paid 10 percent of salaried employees may be denied job restoration to prevent substantial and grievous economic injury to the employer.

- The law excludes any person employed at a worksite with fewer than 50 employees.

- Employee rights are enforceable through civil actions. Actions must be brought not later than 2 years after the date of the last event constituting the alleged violation, or within 3 years of the last event if the violation is willful.

- Complaints about violations of the law are filed with the Department of Labor's Employment Standards Administration (ESA). Inquiries should be directed to local offices of the Wage and Hour Division, ESA.

- The Act does not supersede any State or local law, collective bargaining agreement, or employment benefit plan providing greater employee family leave rights, nor does it diminish the capacity to adopt more generous family leave policies.

- The law became effective August 5, 1993.[1]

---

1. Facts on Working Women, Women's Bureau, U.S. Department of Labor, No. 93-1, March 1993

ALSO FROM BLUE POINT BOOKS

He said, "I don't see why you can't check your voicemail while you're on your honeymoon."

THE MEN AT THE OFFICE

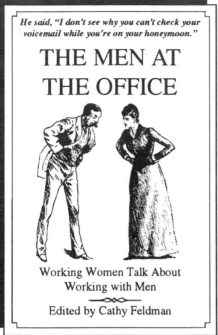

Working Women Talk About
Working with Men

Edited by Cathy Feldman

"I don't know how any family makes it on one income any more."

I WORK TOO

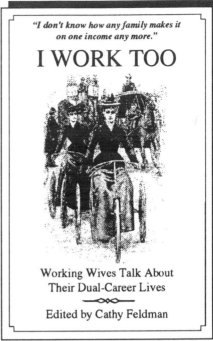

Working Wives Talk About
Their Dual-Career Lives

Edited by Cathy Feldman

The Men At The Office is the second book in Cathy Feldman's series based on her interviews with working women. This time she asked what it's like to work with men. Sometimes hilarious, sometimes outrageous, always right on target, you won't want to miss *The Men At The Office.*
ISBN 1-883423-02-3, $9.95

I Work Too looks at the realities of trying to cope with dual-career lives in the high-pressure 90s. Packed with humor and insights taken directly from interviews with working wives, information, and experts' opinions, *I Work Too* delivers page after page of reassurance that we can make it work.
ISBN 1-883423-05-8, $9.95

Two Years Without Sleep, The Men At The Office, and *I Work Too* can be ordered directly from Blue Point Books. Visa© and MasterCard© accepted.

To order call toll free: **1-800-858-1058**

For information about purchasing our books in quantity for your company or organization, please contact:

Blue Point Books
P.O. Box 91347, Santa Barbara, CA 93109 • 805-965-2635